Can the Keto diet beat Alzheimer's?

The latest available scientific research clearly explained for you to take action and help save the brain of your loved one

Juan L Aguirre

CureByKeto

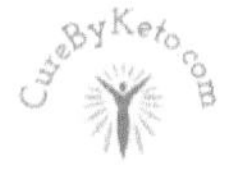

In loving memory of my late paternal grandmother "Abuelita China" (Eva Villafaña), may God have her in the most immense Glory.

CONTENTS

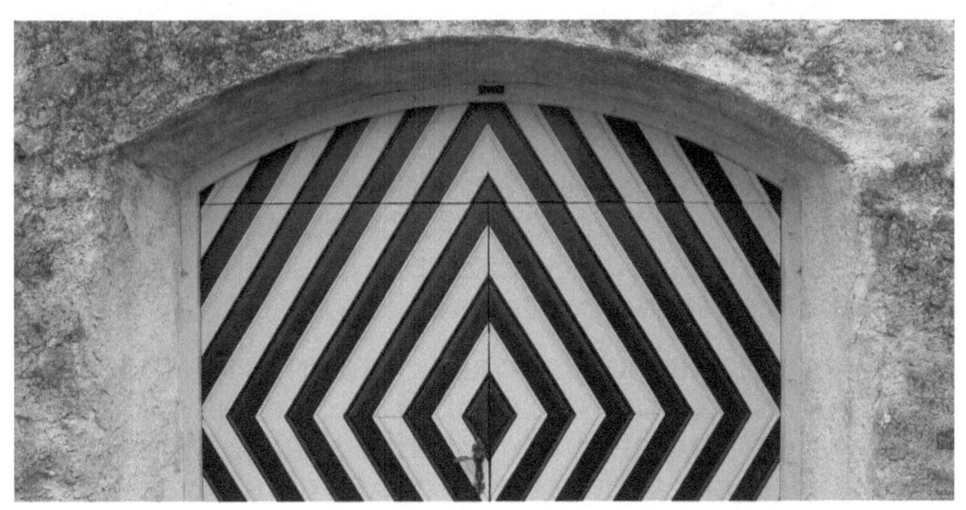

DISCLAIMER

NOTHING IN THIS BOOK OR ANY ELECTRONIC OR OTHER TYPE OF COMMUNICATION FROM US NEITHER CONSTITUTES OR REPLACES MEDICAL ADVICE, THE READER MUST CONSULT ALL HIS/HER HEALTH CARE PROFESSIONALS BEFORE ATTEMPTING ANY TREATMENT OR THERAPY CHANGE. THIS WRITING SIMPLY CONSISTS IN A RECOMPILATION, INFORMATION SELECTION AND EDITION OF FREELY AVAILABLE INFORMATION FROM THE INTERNET AND OTHER PUBLICLY AVAILABLE SOURCES, AND AS SUCH IT IS NOT INTENDED TO REPRESENT SCIENTIFIC OR MEDICAL FACTS WHICH ARE STILL UNDER RESEARCH AND VALIDATION BY THE SCIENTIFIC AND MEDICAL COMMUNITY, PROPER CAUTION IS FULLY ADVISED. FOR QUESTIONS PLEASE CONTACT *ADMIN@CUREBYKETO.COM*, AUSTIN TX, USA, THANK YOU

THIS BOOK USE SUGGESTION

WE SUGGEST YOU READ THIS BOOK, COVER TO COVER AND DO ADDITIONAL RESEARCH OF YOUR OWN AND THEN GIFT ANOTHER COPY OF THIS PUBLICATION TO YOUR MD AND/OR THERAPIST FOR HER TO VALIDATE AND DEFINE DEFINITIVE TREATMENT OPTIONS AND CHANGES, IF ANY.

AT THE END OF THIS BOOK A SERIES OF SCIENTIFIC REFERENCES AND LINKS HAVE BEEN INCLUDED TO FACILITATE STARTING / CONTINUING A MORE SERIOUS PROFESSIONAL ANALYSIS BY THE INTERESTED READER AND/OR QUALIFIED PARTIES.

△△△

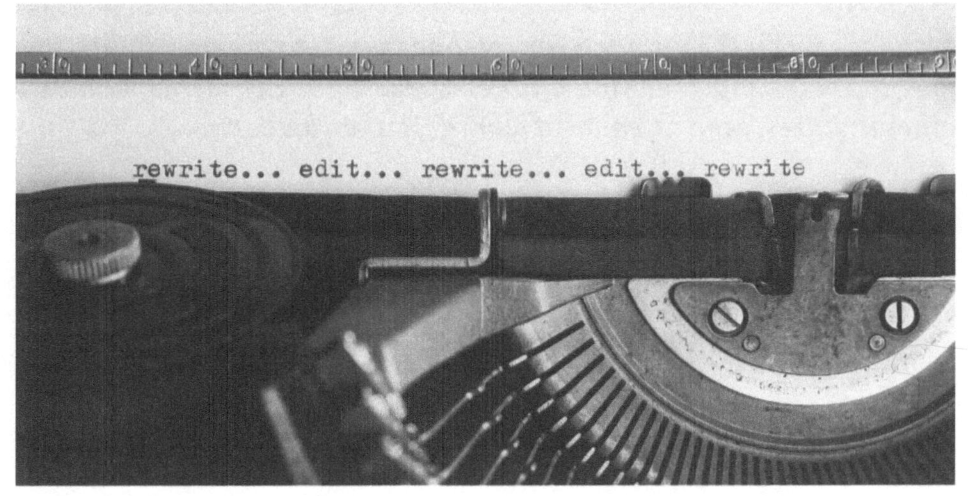

ABOUT THE AUTHORS

Juan L. Aguirre
Juan is a technology-based venture serial entrepreneur, founder and chief-editor of *Amoketo.com* a leading Ketogenic diet social media, community and information resource in Spanish, with dozens of thousands followers worldwide and still growing exponentially. A serious and informed health and fitness professional, obtained his nutritionist certificate in 2019, from the *University of Wageningen*, Netherlands . Avid trail runner, hiker and mountain biker, travels constantly, calls home both Austin TX, and Mexico City.

Jorge Valenzuela, M.D.
Jorge is a renown Medical Doctor (M.D.) writer, translator, devoted and diligent academic researcher. Jorge validated and edited most of this book original material for accuracy and improving its scientific base.

You may reach the authors, for personalized Keto programs with follow up (both in person and online), speaking engagements, and any other inquires, send an email at admin@curebyketo.com

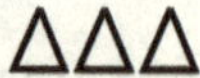

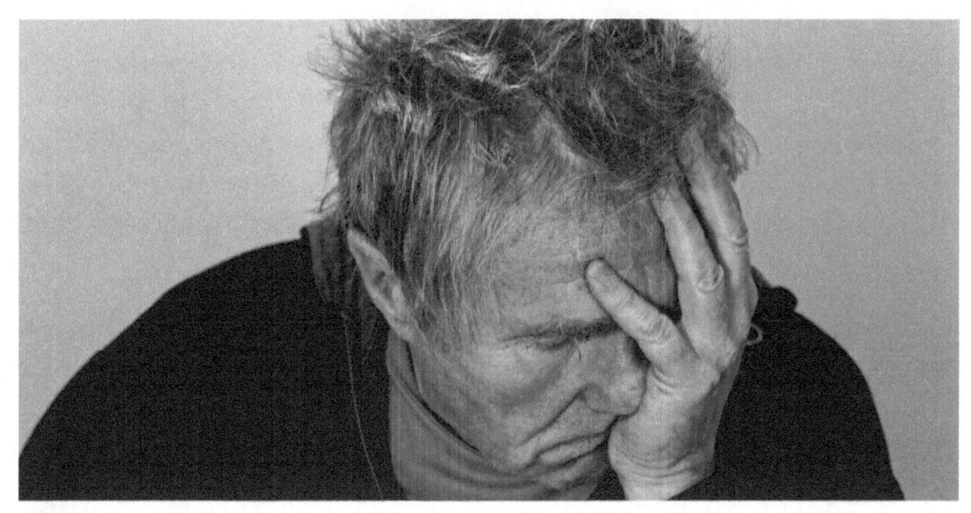

ABSTRACT

The Ketogenic diet has gained popularity in recent years as a dietary plan based on a meal plan with a very low proportion of carbohydrates and a high proportion of fats that can help to accelerate fat burning, that is, less bread, grains and sugars, and more meats and fatty foods.

The name "Keto" comes from the fact that this diet makes it so the body produces a substance called ketones, which is created whenever blood sugar is low and another source of energy is needed.

This book will focus on the effects of a Ketogenic Diet on the treatment and prevention of Alzheimer's Disease, a very well-known disease with a high prevalence in elderly people with an important effect on lifestyle and life expectancy.

First, we will look at what Alzheimer's Disease is and what causes it, as well as the clinical manifestations it has and the repercussion these symptoms have on the patient. After that, we will review some information regarding the role a Keto Diet plays in Alzheimer's Disease, and the benefits it brings to patients that start this meal plan.

Alzheimer's Disease is a progressive irreversible and chronic neurodegenerative disease that accounts for nearly 60% of the known cases of dementia, that is, of memory loss and behavioral change.

The pathogenesis of Alzheimer's, that is, the start and natural evolution of the disease, is very complex. Several studies have found that the way a Ketogenic diet aids in the treatment of Alzheimer's disease is by protecting other brain cells not affected by Alzheimer's, by protecting against the aggregation of more beta-amyloid plaques, and by functioning as an alternative source of fuel for the brain that is not affected by the disease.

A Ketogenic diet is beneficial for patients with Alzheimer's, and adding it into your treatment plan, or that of your patients or relatives, can be beneficial to your or their wellbeing, by being a therapy that allows for cognitive improvement, general wellbeing, and a better lifestyle.

△△△

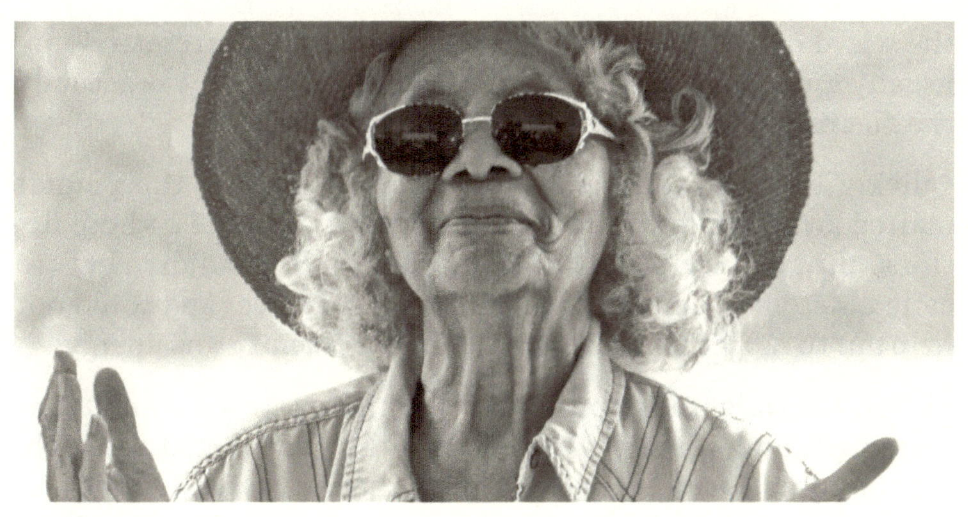

PREFACE

One of my lifetime's more painful memories is to have seen my grandmother suffer many years from Alzheimer's disease until she died when I was still a little kid. That affected me terribly as I loved her dearly and kept in my hearth lots of beautiful memories with her during my early growth years, she was in fact as like a second mother to me.

As it pertains to this book, my story starts 5 years ago, after being overweight most of my life, and exhausted of trying pretty much everything and every diet fad available, in a very desperate state and already with considerable self-image problems, I stumbled upon an intriguing book titled *"Why we get fat"* from Dr. Gary Taubes (2011) and quickly devoured it in few days of intense reading and parallel online research, about all things related to the wierd diet of low carbohydrates, moderate protein and -unusually enough- high fat. (so called good- fats) That was actually the diet called "Ketogenic Diet" or simply "Keto".

Quickly I started following it and to my surprise the pounds melted away in a few months, and contrary to some bad predictions, after a quick period of "body fuel- change" adjustment (so called "Keto flu" for a reason) I felt better than ever and could not help but to notice a much enhanced mental acuity and energy.

I loved the weight loss, but I was very more intrigued about the seemingly brain benefits of the Keto diet, so started researching the topic extensively with much interest, what I found out shocked me much. As the most documented origin of the Keto diet was as an intended treatment of Epilepsy patients, taking place in the Mayo clinic during the 1920's, it was a treatment pioneered by late Dr Wilder, (see http://bit.ly/2KKFuCp) as conclusion it was found that the "ketones", which are the byproduct of lipid breakdown whilst restricting carbohydrates in a Keto diet, have in fact some very scientifically-proven beneficial properties related to neurological heath.

How the heck these great and very simple brain-enhancing properties have escaped from public knowledge for ages? It was obvious to me, in my own personal experience, that ketones provided an incredible mental energy source, and could have much wider brain benefits that just treating Epilepsy, I wondered what other neurological conditions this could be applied for?

I decided to research even more the topic, probably I could find some literature and solid scientific backing for using the Keto diet as auxiliary treatment for other diseases, probably even for Alzheimer.

This book is the final result of that research which took place during most of 2019.

I would like this to become a sort of remembrance and homage for my very dear late "abuela" (grandma), and a means to sending her my deepest love wherever she is.

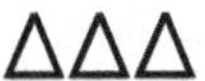

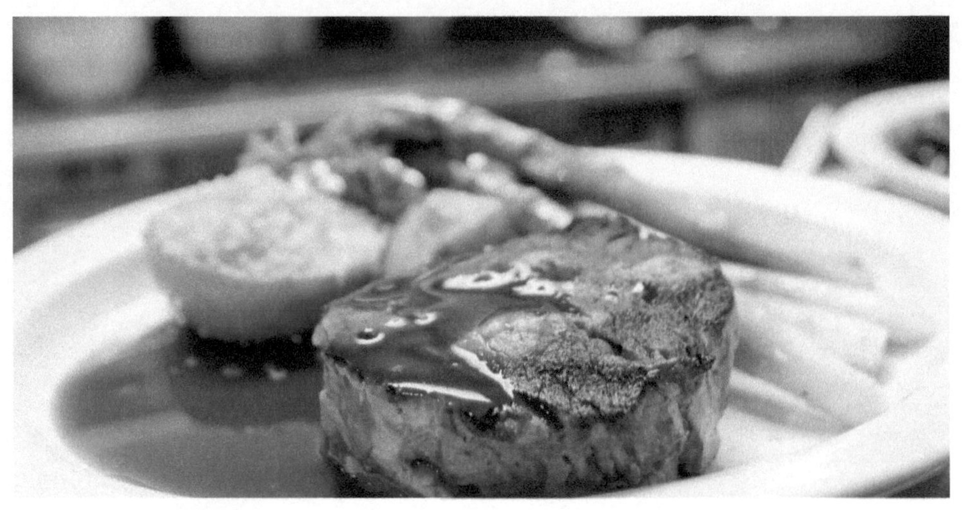

INTRODUCTION

What is a Ketogenic diet? What is Alzheimer's Disease? What is the best way to treat this very serious disease? Is there anything else I can do or something I can add to my treatment plan to further improve my health? Can a Ketogenic diet really help to treat Alzheimer's?

Questions like these are constantly asked, and most of the times the answers to them are found in non-reliable sources, or with close to zero information to back it up, often leaving the readers with a sense of loss, disbelief or doubt.

Ketogenic diets are frequently recommended to people as means to easily lose fat and weight, but they are being recommended more and more as treatment options for patients with serious degenerative and incapacitating diseases such as Alzheimer's,

Parkinson's, ALS, and epilepsy, to improve their general well-being and improve their lifestyle. But how good are they actually?

WHAT IS THE KETOGENIC DIET?

The Ketogenic diet has gained popularity in recent years as a dietary plan based on a meal plan with a very low proportion of carbohydrates and a high proportion of fats that can help to accelerate fat burning, that is, less bread, grains, legumes and sugars, and more meats, green leafy vegetables , and fatty foods.

The name "Keto" comes from the fact that this diet makes it so the body produces a substance called ketones, which are created whenever blood sugar is low and another source of energy is needed, usually using protein and fat as a source, which are taken in by the liver to be transformed into these ketones.

After they leave the liver, they can go to different parts of the body to work as a fuel source, such as the brain, which requires a lot of energy daily to work properly that can be obtained from sugar; a fact unknown to many is that even though the brain represents only 5% of the total body weight, it consumes up to 30% of the available energy in our bodies to be constantly working.

As it has been recently discovered, the brain can also acquire fuel and energy from ketones; with this information in hand it is easier to understand how a Ketogenic diet can aid in fat burning: when your body starts running low on sugar, it switches to using fat as an energy source, by converting it into ketones without needing to go through fasting or unneeded hunger.

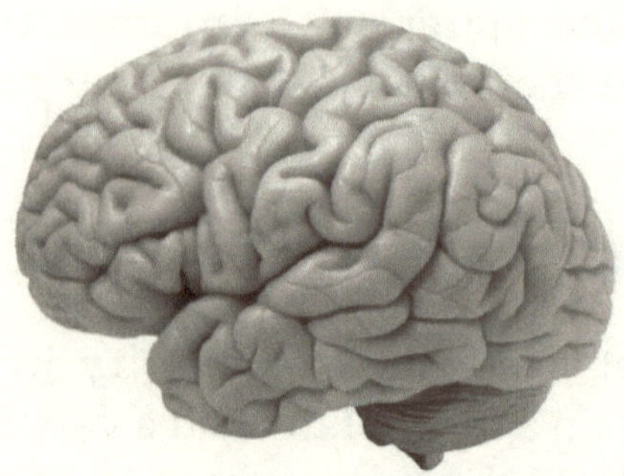

IMG 1.- *The brain represents only 5%of the total body weight, but it uses up to 30% of all he available energy, which is usually obtained from fuel sources such as glucose; if the energy supply to the brain is interrupted, millions of cells can rapidly die, causing serious negative effects on the mood, thinking capacity, memory, and overall health of the patient.*

In the past, this same approach of resorting to the metabolism of fats was achieved by long hours of fasting, as a matter of fact, there are a couple of articles available on the history of the Ketogenic diet that tell the story of fasting used as a method of treating epilepsy and other seizure-related diseases, which proved to be useful for these patients but hard on the body on the long run.

In the past, this same approach of resorting to the metabolism of fats was achieved by long hours of fasting, as a matter of fact, there are a couple of articles available on the history of the Ketogenic diet that tell the story of fasting used as a method of treating epilepsy and other seizure-related diseases, which proved to be useful for these patients but hard on the body on the long run.

In 1921 another article proposed that acetone and beta-hydroxybutyric acid (both of which are ketones) which are normally produced during fasting periods, can also be created by switching and sticking to a low carb and high fat diet, which also proved beneficial to the same seizure patients who showed dramatic improvement in their condition, thus coming into existence the 'Ketogenic Diet'.

Several articles can be found online regarding the benefits that having a Ketogenic diet can have for you, and much more focus has been given to this topic by the medical and scientific community that have directed their focus towards finding out if this 'Keto Diet' can be beneficial for people with severe and incapacitating diseases, including neurological diseases such as Alzheimer disease, epilepsy, Parkinson's, autism, metabolic and cardiovascular diseases such as hypertension, diabetes, dyslipidemia, and autoimmune diseases such as rheumatoid arthritis, systemic erythematous lupus and osteoarthritis.

Also, a Ketogenic diet allows your body to go into a state of ketosis, that is the presence of ketones in your body, usually only doable after long periods of starvation; this in turn helps with lowering blood sugar, which when constantly high, as in patients with diabetes, can cause damage to your brain.

OTHER DISEASES THE KETO DIET MAY BENEFIT

Other neurological diseases win which Keto Diet has been studied as a possible therapeutic tool with promising results are:

- **Seizures (Epilepsy)**
- **Parkinson's Disease**
- **Migraines**
- **Depression**
- **Anxiety**
- **Cancer**
- **Traumatic brain injury**

Other positive effects regarding the general well-being of patients that have been linked to the use of a Keto Diet have been:

- **Reducing inflammation;** if inflammation is constantly present over a long period of time, it can increase the risk of having serious diseases such as cardiovascular disease, heart attack or a stroke, kidney disease, and cancer, as well as being an important risk factor for chronic diseases such as Alzheimer's disease.

• **Less oxidative stress,** which allows for less damage to the body and DNA, decreasing the risk of developing heart, brain and kidney problems.

• **Balancing glutamate and GABA**, which are molecules related to the activating / inhibiting activities of various cell systems in the body, like the ones that occur during brain processes and neuronal activity.

• **Favoring Omega 3,** which is an important molecule related to the metabolism of fats and oils in our body, reducing the risk of cardiovascular disease or other fat-related problems.

• **Increasing BDNF** (Brain Derived Neurotropic Factor) production, a protein linked with neuronal growth and survival, that is very important for the growth and development of the nervous system.

The studies researching these effects have shown promising preliminary results, which has gained lots of attention from the medical community in hopes of being implemented as a therapy.

This book will focus on the effects of a Ketogenic Diet on the treatment and prevention of Alzheimer's Disease (AD), a very well-known disease with a high prevalence in elderly people with an important effect on lifestyle and life expectancy.

First, we will look at what Alzheimer's Disease is and what causes it, as well as the clinical manifestations it has and the repercussion these symptoms have on the patient. After that, we will review some information regarding the role a Keto Diet plays in Alzheimer's Disease, and the benefits it brings to patients that start this meal plan. (More information about how to actually do this and implementation suggestions in pages which follow)

A lot of interest has gone towards researching the therapeutic effects of a Keto diet, which is one of the main reasons this book has been written, as well as being a reliable source of information regarding this topic in lieu of the wide array of unreliable sources available on the internet and other media outlets.

THE KETO DIET FOOD PYRAMID

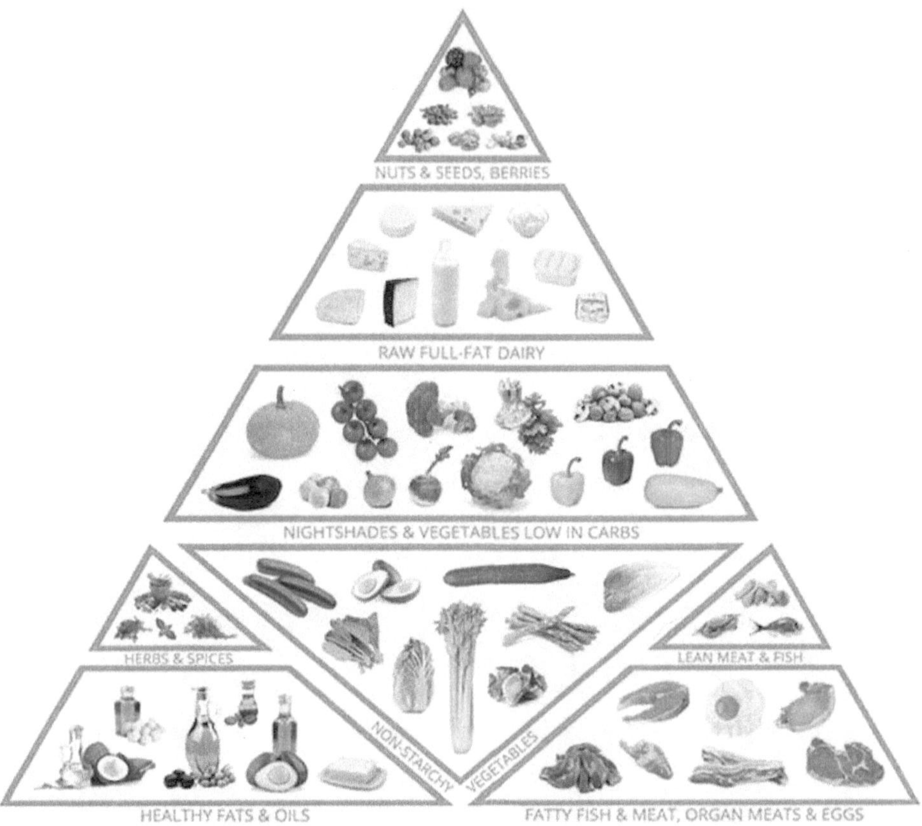

AVOID: *Bread, cookies, sweets, sugars, cereals, legumes, starchy vegetables (like potatoes, carrots), rice, beans, soy, most other grains and almost all fruits (i.e. strawberries are OK).*

CALORIE INTAKE: *70% from good fats, 25% from protein, 5% from Carbohydrates.* (of your suggested daily requirements)

ΔΔΔ

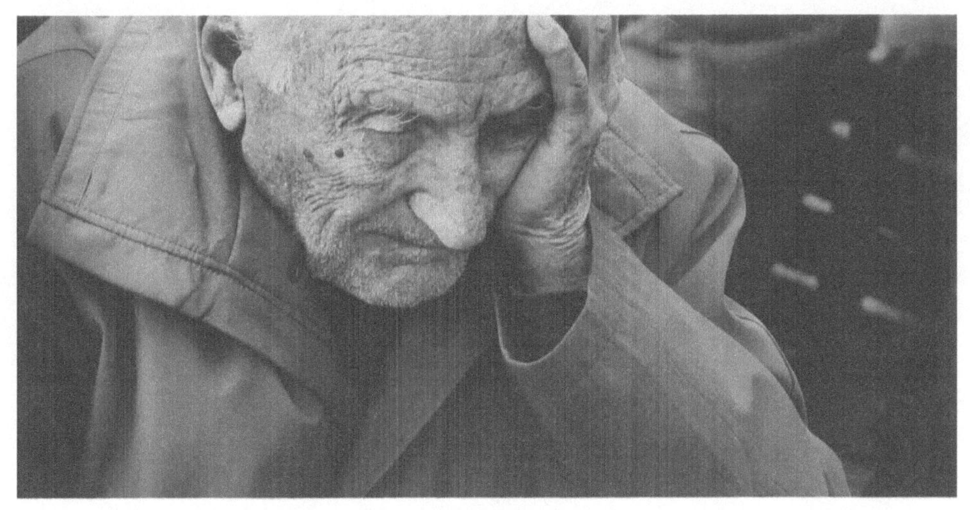

THE ALZHEIMER'S DISEASE

The authors of this book reviewed hundreds of short articles and videos intending to explain of Alzheimer's in comprehensive, simple and clear terms. That's no question that's a significant challenge because the origins, mechanism and complexity of the disease are huge, and most principles are still under very active research and sometimes even heated discussion. The following movie from the National Institute of Aging (USA), is possibly the best introductory material for quickly understanding this terrible public health problem.

MOVIE EXPLAINING THE ALZHEIMER'S DISEASE (AD)

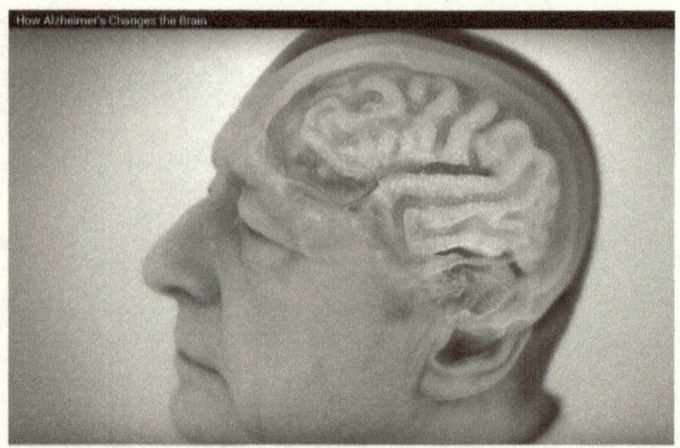

Video 1: *This 4-minute video shows how Alzheimer's disease changes the brain and looks at promising ideas to treat and prevent the disease. CREDIT: National Institute of Aging (USA). To watch in paperback book go to http://bit.ly/2ShnW2Z*

Alzheimer's Disease is a progressive irreversible and chronic neurodegenerative disease that accounts for nearly 60% of the known cases of dementia, that is, of memory loss and behavioral change, and it represents the sixth major cause of death in the US; however, some studies suggest it may be one of the three main causes of death in the country, urging for more effective treatment options for this disease.

It tends to affect people older than 65 years, with a much higher prevalence after 85 years, and the main risk factors that have been linked to having or not Alzheimer's Disease are: old age, having relatives that have or had Alzheimer's or Parkinson's, having hypertension, diabetes or other psychiatric alterations, smoking, Down Syndrome, or having a background of previous head trauma.

Diabetes mellitus type II (usually shortened as DM-II), in which there is an important resistance to the effects of insulin, the substance in charge of making our muscles and cells capable of taking in the sugar we eat in our diets, is a disease that has been suggested to have a very strong link with Alzheimer's Disease.

In DM-II, the effects of insulin on the body's cells is decreased, causing a rise in the blood sugar levels due to the inability of the cells to take it in; these higher sugar levels can cause very serious complications such as vascular disease, heart problems, eye problems that can end up in blindness, and, as it has been recently studied, Alzheimer's disease.

As we will see, one key factor in the development of Alzheimer's Disease is a change in the uptake and usage of energy by the brain, which is already altered in diabetic patients, further contributing to the development and progression of Alzheimer's. Some other factors that have been proposed as to be linked with this disease are nutritional deficiencies, mostly deficiencies in vitamin E, C, B6 and B12, and the use of certain drugs and substances such as alcohol or recreational drugs.

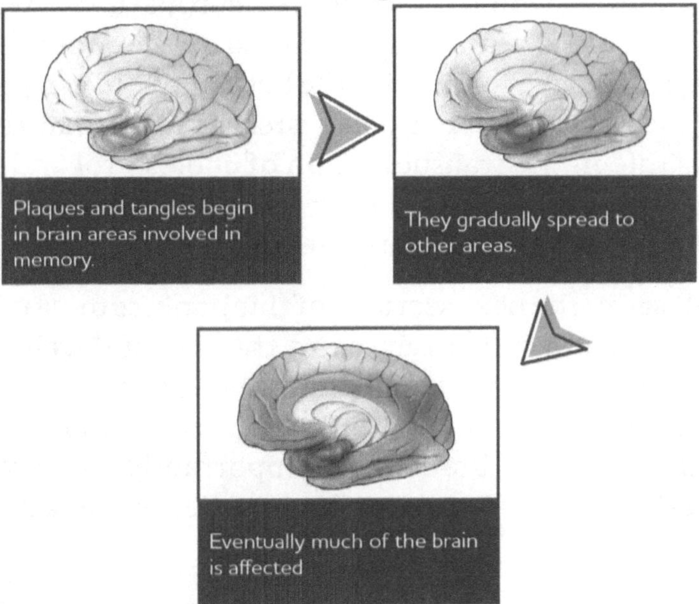

IMG 2.- *How Alzheimer's spreads in the brain. CREDIT: National Institute of Aging (USA)*

The pathogenesis of Alzheimer's, that is, the start and natural evolution of the disease, is very complex. Several articles have been written that try to pinpoint the exact cause for this disease, however, none has been conclusive, leading to a wide array of theories that try to explain the specific cause for Alzheimer's.

One of the most accepted theories is that a glue-like substance called Beta-amyloid, a peptide produced from another protein called 'Amyloid Precursor Protein', first deposits itself in the hippocampus, the brain's area that is mainly related to memory, followed by the alteration of a protein called 'tau' located in the microtubules of the neurons, that is, the scaffolding that helps the cells keep their shape, leading to the formation of tau conglomerates that are more commonly called 'neurofibrillary tangles'.

These two alterations together cause changes in the neuronal transport system, which then leads to neuronal and synapsis loss that produces the disease's cognitive and memory deterioration. However, it has been found that the beta-amyloid can be present in other diseases, as well as being present in normal situations due to its role in the transportation of cholesterol and the activation of enzymes, so further research needs to be conducted to pinpoint the exact cause of this disease.

As we will see in the next sections of this book, some studies have pointed out that a factor related to the risk of developing Alzheimer's, and the speed at which the disease progresses once it has established itself, is the deficit in energy uptake (mostly glucose) in several areas of the brain (more importantly those related to Alzheimer's), in other words the brain suffers from lack of nutrients.

This occurs with age, which leads to a degenerative process that further increases the risk of having this disease; we will go further into this matter in the following sections, as well as the role that ketones have in decreasing the risk of having Alzheimer and in slowing down the progression of the disease.

The build-up of these protein plaques in the blood vessels that go to the brain, and in the main areas of the brain that are responsible of memory, alter the energy supply of the brain, causing it to receive less fuel than what a normal brain would receive, leading to the death of a huge amount of neurons, thus causing the brain shrinking and deterioration characteristic of Alzheimer's, which leads to memory and cognitive problems.

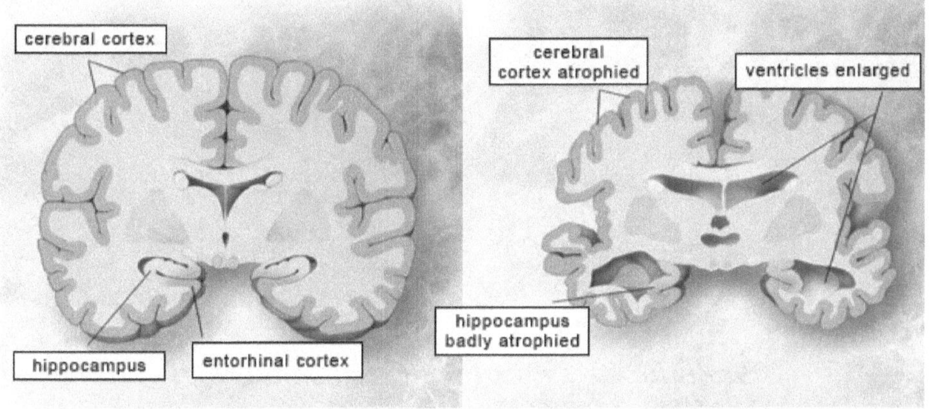

IMG 3.- *Healthy brain at the left, and shrunk and atrophied Alzheimer's patient brain at the right. CREDIT: Garrondo*

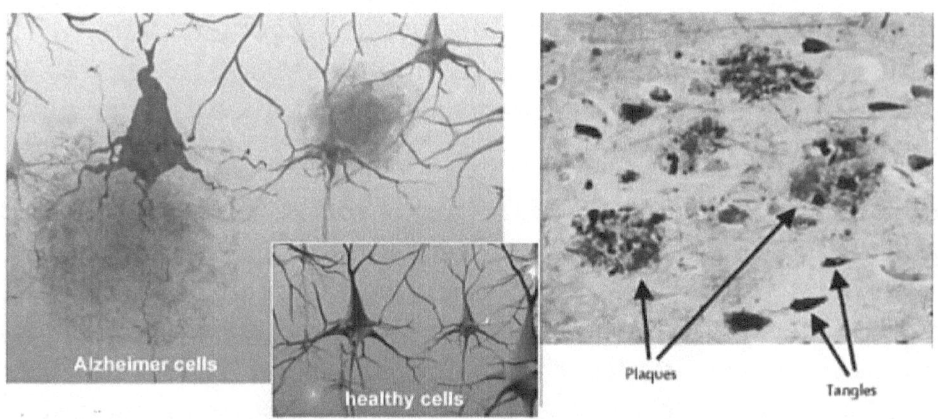

IMG 4.- *Progression of Alzheimer's disease attacking the brain cells (neurons), showing formation of "amyloid plaques" (left) as well as "tau proteins" buildup (right). CREDIT: alz.org & The Lancet, Blennow K, MJ de León, and H Zatterberg*

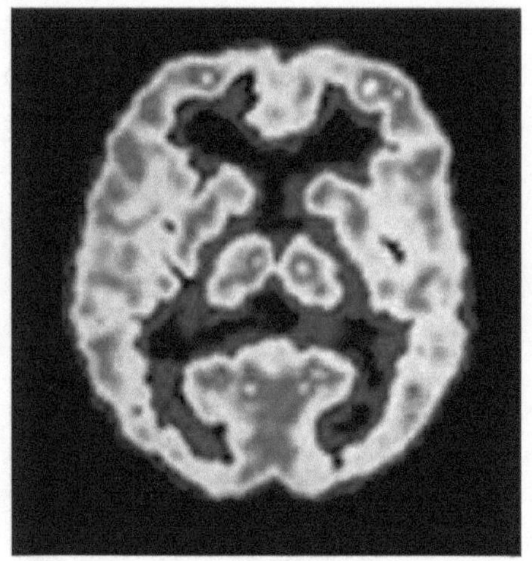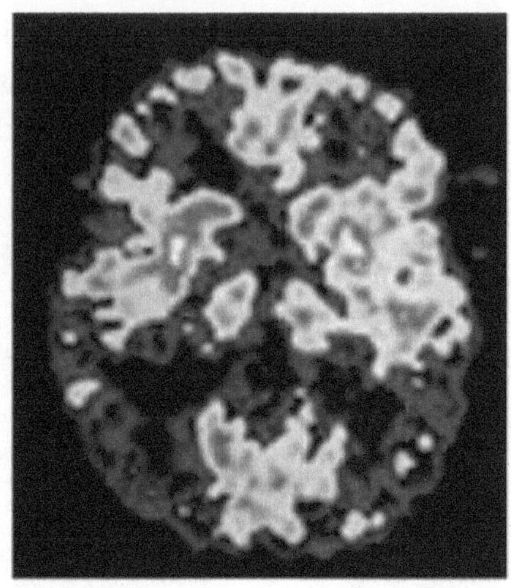

IMG 5.- Left brain healthy glucose (nutrient) uptake, right brain decreased uptake (lacking sufficient nutrients, hence causing massive braincell death). CREDIT: Dan Krtoz. "New clue in the search to predict Alzheimer's", December 2008.

The clinical course of Alzheimer's paints a very well-known picture, with patients that develop memory problems that with time tend to become more serious and incapacitating, as well as developing behavioral and cognitive alterations, such as changes in vocabulary and mood.

Alzheimer's is like a snowball that is rolled from the top of a mountain; at first, it starts as a very minor inconvenience with occasional memory problems such as remembering a name, a date or a fact, but later evolves into a severe disease with near to full dependency, usually leading to the death of the patient after 3 to 10 years after the initial diagnosis. The disease's progression has been divided into 4 stages:

• **Preclinical** – a normal patient with no symptoms, but detectable alterations in the brain.

• **Mild Alzheimer's** – a patient with mild memory problems, changes in mood and personality with a tendency towards anxiety, and confusion.

• **Moderate Alzheimer's** – a patient with a more severe memory deterioration, with a difficulty to maintain focus, organize, and apply logic, with a more intense anxiety that couples with hallucinations and delirium.

• **Severe Alzheimer's -** a patient with the symptoms mentioned before, but with a rise in intensity to the point of making the patient dependable of someone else's care.

Several different therapies have been developed and tested in order to both prevent and treat cases of Alzheimer's, but none has proven to be 100% effective in stopping the disease's progression, most tend to just ameliorate the symptoms.

DRUGS USED TO ATTEMPT ALZHEIMER'S TREATMENT

The most common type of drug used are acetylcholinesterase inhibitors (ACI), such as donepezil, galantamine and rivastigmine, but these cause a lot of secondary effects, primarily nausea, vomit, diarrhea, pain, weight loss, alterations in sleep, incontinency and extrapyramidal symptoms (loss of balance, falls, etc.), and they are not recommended in patients with heart problems, lung problems such as CPOD, epilepsy, hypotension, gastric ulcers or asthma.

Another kind of drug therapy commonly used are glutaminergic modulators, such as memantine, usually used in moderate to severe cases due to its efficiency in monotherapy, that is, being used on its own. However, this drug also comes with its fair share of secondary effects, such as constipation, lightheadedness, insomnia, hypertension, anxiety and confusion.

Most of the drugs used nowadays to treat Alzheimer's Disease are mostly used for palliative means, that is, to try and control and reduce the severity of the symptoms as much as possible to try and keep the quality of life as high as possible, however, this does not mean the disease is being cured or progression is stopped.

As you can see, the usual treatment of Alzheimer's requires a long list of medications, that need to be changed or modified constantly in order to be as effective as they can be for the patient, and still, the disease tends to continue its path and deterioration continues to exacerbate

That is why a huge effort has been made in order to find alternative therapies that can help stop the progression of symptoms in these patients with the least amount of side effects possible.

One of these therapies has been the implementation of a Ketogenic diet into the Alzheimer patient's treatment plan; several studies have been conducted where the effects of this diet on Alzheimer's have been documented, as well as the possible benefits switching to this plan can have on preventing and treating the disease.

△△△

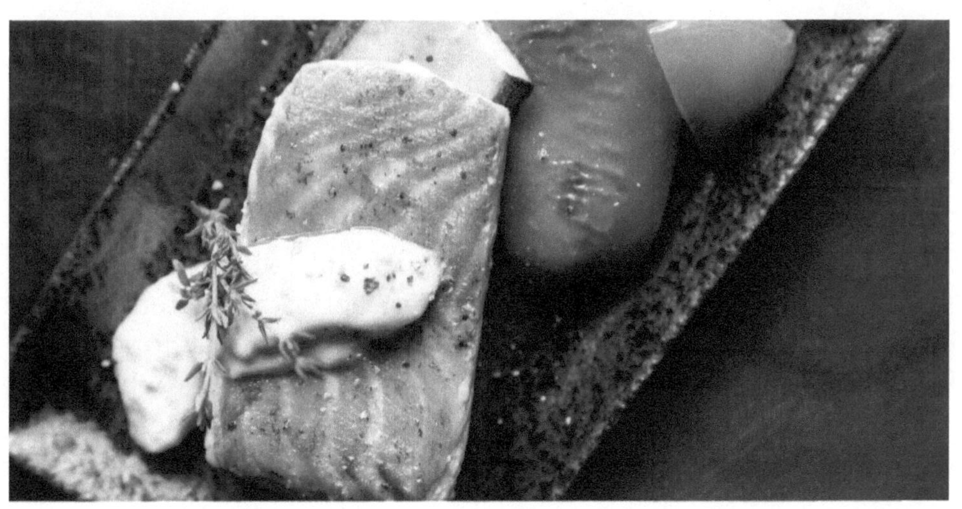

EFFECT OF THE KETO
DIET ON ALZHEIMER'S

Most of these studies have found that the way a ketogenic diet aids in the treatment of Alzheimer's disease is by protecting other brain cells not affected by Alzheimer's, by stopping the aggregation of more beta-amyloid plaques, and by functioning as an alternative source of fuel for the brain that is not affected by the nutrient-blocking effect of the disease.

In one study performed in 2018 (7), it was shown that a ketogenic diet reduces the neuronal hyperexcitability normally present in early Alzheimer's disease by increasing the production of GABA, an inhibitory neurotransmitter that normally slows down or interrupts neuronal activity, as well as by regulating mitochondrial metabolism by increasing mitochondrial biogenesis in key parts of the brain, favoring the regulation of calcium and ROS (reactive oxygen species) production.

This means that by adopting a ketogenic diet, Alzheimer's patients help their brain produce beneficial substances such as GABA, which stops the altered brain activity related to Alzheimer's, and regulate the function of their mitochondria, an important metabolic regulator, inside the brain-cells, which participates in the production and elimination of beneficial and prejudicial substances for the brain.

Another study published in 2016 (8) aimed to investigate the effects of an inefficient glucose uptake during aging and its relationship with Alzheimer's disease as an important risk factor. As we have mentioned before, the brain uses a huge amount of energy on a daily basis, which it normally tends to obtain mainly from glucose.

However, with age, the ability for the brain to uptake glucose from the bloodstream to keep its normal functions tends to become worse and worse, leading to having some areas of the brain receive a lesser amount of energy than they need, creating a vicious cycle based around brain glucose hypometabolism, (getting less amount of nutrients than needed to operate) that favors deterioration and neuronal dysfunction, which increases the risk and speed of progression of Alzheimer's.

KETONES USED AS ALTERNATIVE BRAIN FUEL

In contrast, it was found that brain ketone uptake is not affected by age like glucose, which can be diminished by the presence of the protein plaques we mentioned before, making it harder for the brain to receive fuel and energy, and that a ketone-based diet (Ketogenic diet) can be used in mild-to-moderate cases of Alzheimer's to compensate for the deficient glucose uptake just like it normally happens during periods of starvation due to the ability of ketones to avoid the protein plaques and provide fuel and energy to the brain just as well as glucose.

This fact has been demonstrated in various clinical trials where patients with Alzheimer's disease show improvement in cognitive outcomes after being started with a Ketogenic diet with 20-70 g/day of triglycerides or ketone esters, that is, a diet with a higher fat concentration. Studies like this push the need for the development of therapeutic strategies that aim towards correcting the underlying fuel supply problem related to Alzheimer that has been shown to increase the risk of having the disease, as well as accelerating the progression of the clinical course.

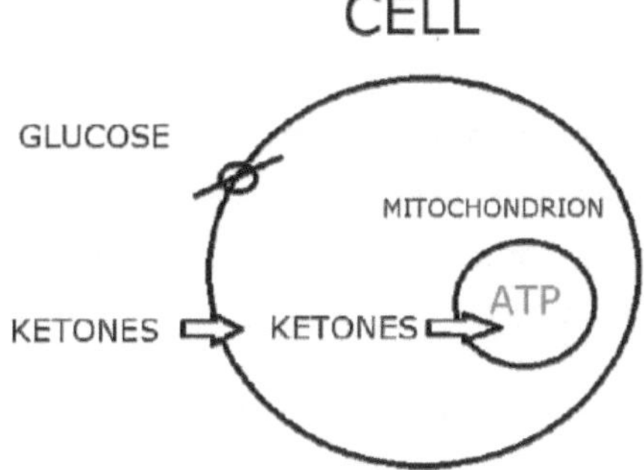

IMG 6.- Glucose which is the "typical" brain fuel gets blocked by Alzheimer's progress, but ketones, an alternative source of energy generated during the Ketogenic diet, are not, therefore are able to reach inside of the brain-cells (neurons) to be converted into ATP (by cell's internal mitochondrion micro-organs) which is the final source of energy for the cells to survive and function in a healthy manner.

In a study conducted in 2018 (10), the feasibility of a Ketogenic diet on patients with Alzheimer's Disease was investigated; in this study, patients were given a 3 month Ketogenic diet, during which they were tested for blood and urine ketones, as well as having their cognitive status tested through the Mini-Mental State Examination (a tool usually used to assess the cognitive status of a patient when delirium, dementia or Alzheimer's are suspected) before and after the diet.

This study was based as well on the premise presented by the article we described before, where an energy deficit has been linked as a key factor in the pathogenesis and progression of Alzheimer's, promoting the use of a ketone-rich diet as means to allow the brain to maintain its normal energy uptake from a source different than normal sugar / glucose.

After the 3 months of diet, the patients were re-assessed using the Mini-Mental and other tools to evaluate dementia, finding an improvement of up to 100% in their cognitive status, thus forwarding the recommendation of starting Alzheimer's patients on a ketone-rich diet based around higher concentrations of triglycerides and other fats.

Studies and clinical trials are being constantly published regarding the uses and benefits of a Ketogenic diet on patients with Alzheimer's and other neurodegenerative diseases, such as Parkinson's, ALS, and epilepsy.

The general consensus regarding this diet plan is that it is beneficial for this kind of patients, even more so in mild-to-moderate cases, which show a significative improvement in their general cognitive status, mood, and general wellbeing, thus allowing for a slower clinical progression, milder symptoms, and a better lifestyle for the patient.

You can discuss the possibility of starting a Ketogenic diet with your doctor, as well as getting more professional advice from a certified nutritionist or dietician, in order to perfectly establish the contents and portions of the diet plan, as well as scheduling for check ups and follow ups; however, it is important to keep in mind that every case differs from one another, so not all Alzheimer's patients will be treated the same way; always seek assistance from a medical professional before making decisions regarding your treatment or the treatment of someone else.

As initial guidance, in the next chapter we include some tentative recommendations about how to approach the change of diet for an AD patient, hope this helps as the startup point to help you define the best plan

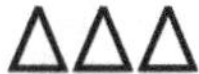

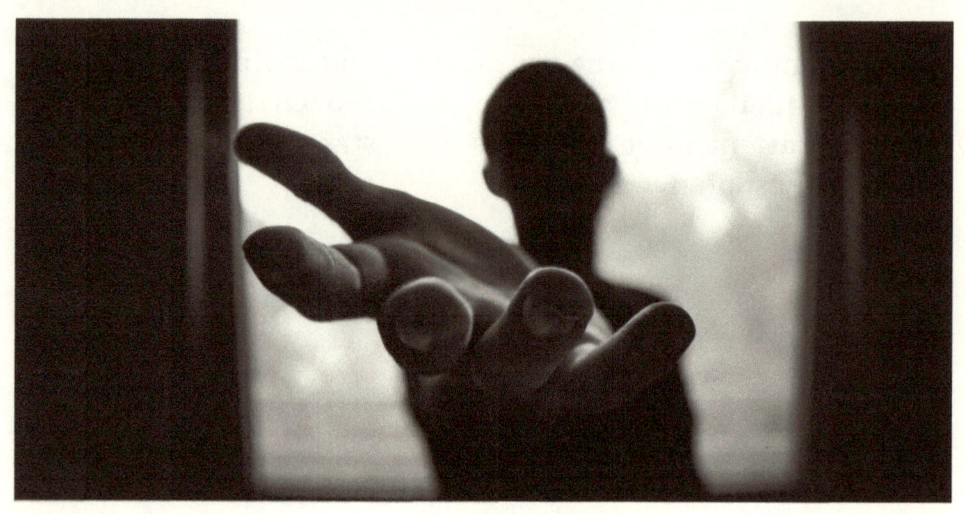

ACTION STEPS AND CONSIDERATIONS

This book has described already how the Alzheimer's disease (AD) has been scientifically proven to be a metabolic condition, that means a disease related to nutrition, and how the body obtains energy and other elements necessary to survive, repair and grow.

This book has described already how Alzheimer's has been scientifically proven to be (mostly) a metabolic condition, that means a disease related to nutrition, and how the body obtains energy and other elements necessary to survive, repair and grow.

Glucose is the primary energy source for the brain, but it has been found that Ketones, (such as beta-hydroxybutyrate (βOHB) and acetoacetate) which are a byproduct of the Ketogenic diet can supply up to 60% of brain's energy needs, that supply is available and beneficial even to atrophied brain cells, restoring them back quickly from a certain death.

Only 60%, of energy coming from Ketones, could sound not enough but in most patients some glucose metabolization is still going on (specially in early disease stages), therefore Ketones don't need to provide 100% of energy supply for the brain, but only aid as a complement. However many patients will show significant improvement with much less than 60%, even some are able to improve cognitive function with as little as 5 - 10% of additional energy supply.

WAYS TO SUPPLY KETONES TO THE STARVING BRAIN

So far we have discussed the Ketogenic diet, as the primary way to but the body in the metabolic state of "Ketosis" and releasing the body and brain feeding elements called Ketones, such as beta-hydroxybutyrate (βOHB) and acetoacetate. However happily there are alternative or complementary ways to achieve and/or improve or maintain such state trough food supplementation.

Available Keto-related supplements available are "MCT Oil" a dietary supplement made of highly purified coconut and palm oil, and "exogenous ketones" which are supplements products, distributed as mixing powders and pills, produced and commercialized by several well known manufacturers such as "Pruvit", "Ketone", and "Perfect Keto". (you may email the authors for recommendations)

However is important to mention that it has been scientifically proven than supplementation does not mimic all the benefit effects of a real Ketogenic diet, sadly there is nothing (yet) like "Keto in a pill", therefore supplementation should be considered primarily as an "aid" not a replacement in a Ketogenic nutritional therapy.

You may reach, via email, the book authors for suggestions about best, tested and safer Ketogenic supplements available in your market at admin@curebyketo.com

TREATING THE AD PATIENT

In old uncooperative and even belligerent AD patients, often living in assisted living facilities, it could be very challenging to modify any nutritional regimen. Other important consideration is that digestive capacity and performance normally decrease with age, therefore extreme caution needs to be taken whilst changing diet and/or administering nutritional supplements.

Fat and protein digestion for the old secluded AD patient, often becomes difficult, specially coming from many years with a diet abundant in bread, grains and pasta, which is often the case. Also frequently the person could be underweight - therefore becomes essential to avoid fasting (a common practice amongst many Keto enthusiasts) or reduced protein intake.

Potentially MCT oil supplementation along with a well monitored, by your doctor or nutritionist, slow but steadily carbohydrate reduction program, during several months, could result in a sustainable and safe option, worth exploring for some patients. You may possibly like to discuss this with your health care professional and and give it a try. In any case avoid drastic changes.

To find the optimum Ketogenic diet for a particular AD patient, adjustment and experimentation is key, keep an eye in what's working, and do more of it. Often after just a couple of weeks some improved cognition hints could suddenly appear meaning you are headed in the right direction.

Also take in consideration any digestive issues and problems as such discomforts, because if severe, could nullify any achieved positive effect, and make ir difficult to decide continuing making changes.

Our final word of advice is also essential, take in consideration emotional support is very important, always interact with love, care and patience, try to explain whats happening and celebrate any small victories. Create/Improve empathy.

Thanks for reading this book, hope we have being able to communicate our deep enthusiasm and hope for the potential of this complementary AD therapy, and motivated you to play an important role in its development and widespread.

Please keep us posted* about how you have used the information in this book to help improving the life of your loved one.

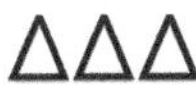

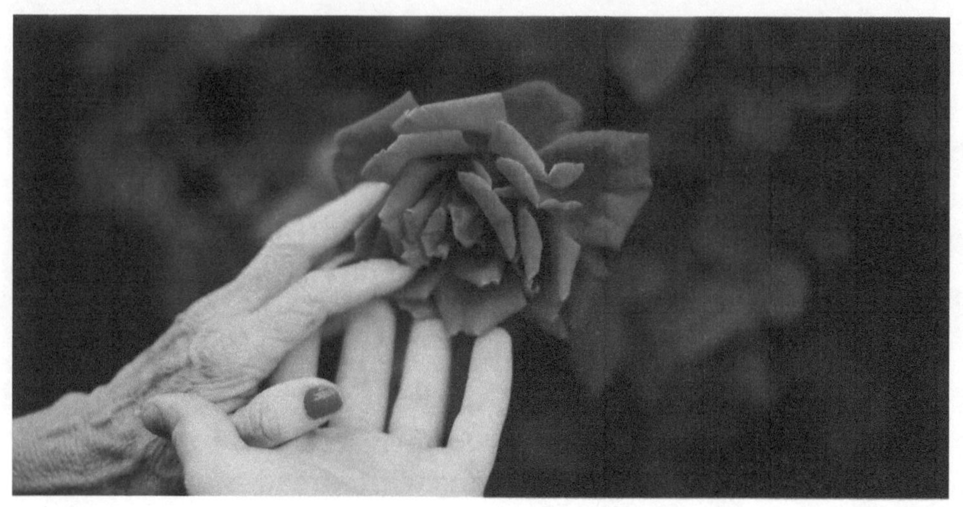

IN CONCLUSION

We have gone through the general aspects of a Ketogenic diet, which we have defined as a diet that consists mostly of fats and protein, with little to none carbohydrates, thus allowing for the production of ketones, an alternative energy source to glucose that is normally produced during starvation periods but that can be created intentionally with a Ketogenic diet.

In several studies, it has been proven that a Ketogenic diet is beneficial to further improve the general wellbeing and improve the clinical conditions of patients affected with chronic or degenerative diseases such as Parkinson's, epilepsy, ALS, and, as we have discussed in this article, Alzheimer's.

Alzheimer's is a very complex disease with a pathogenesis that hasn't been well established yet, but there are a lot of theories available that point towards a degenerative process that affects the neurons and certain parts of the brain (mostly the hippocampus) with the production of altered proteins and protein tangles, probably secondary to the inefficient energy uptake that comes with aging, a process that can be prevented and corrected with a diet rich in ketones, which can pass into the brain and be used as energy just as well as glucose, but without the changes in uptake efficiency related to age like glucose.

Based on this information, several studies were conducted where these hypotheses were tested, and where therapeutic options and proposals were put on trial in order to see how effective they were in treating Alzheimer's; what most of them concluded was that a ketogenic diet improves the cognitive status of patients, as well as decreasing the risk of developing the disease.

A Ketogenic diet is beneficial for patients with Alzheimer's, and adding it into your treatment plan, or that of your patients or relatives, can be beneficial to your or their wellbeing, by being a therapy that allows for cognitive improvement, general wellbeing, and a better lifestyle.

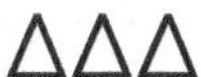

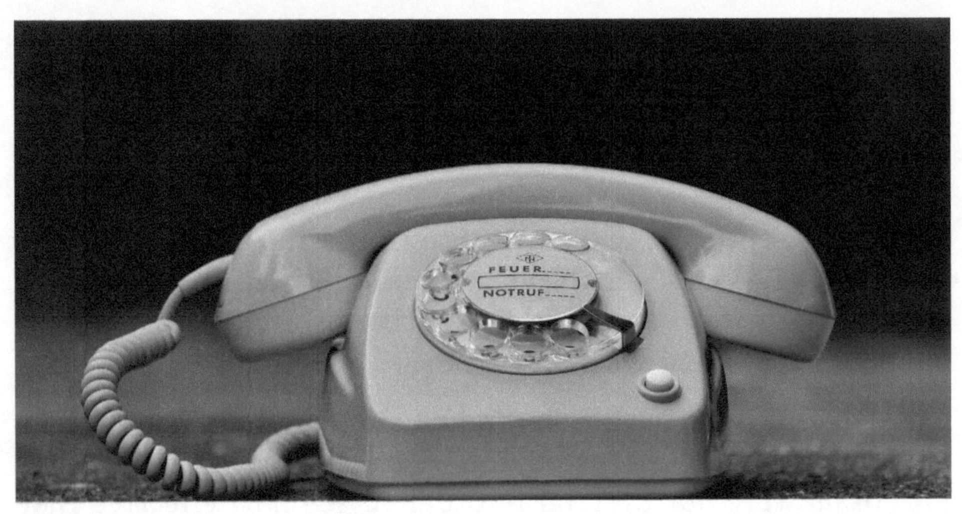

CONTACTING THE AUTHORS

The authors will be happy to hear back from you anytime, for any question, or inquiry, including the following:

• **Volume purchasing of this book** at institutional or discount rates.

• **Quality tested product recomendations** including: supplements, "exogenous ketones", MCT oil, Keto sticks (to detect and measure ketosis), and many others available locally or to be purchased online via approved suppliers.

• **Writing or speaking engagements,** consulting, and research projects, joint ventures and other business oportunities.

Please kindly send an email to admin@curebyketo.com for fast reply. Also contact for feedback or suggestions about this book.

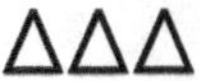

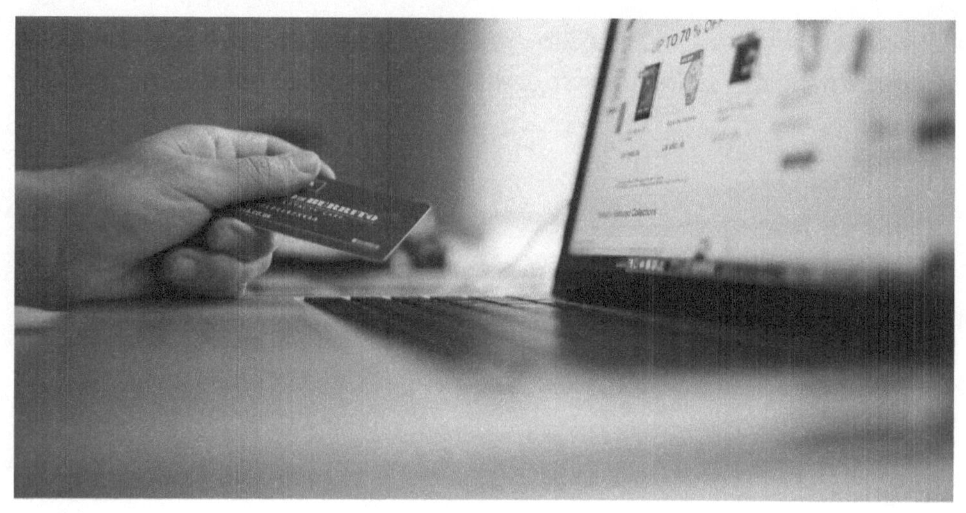

SOME SUGGESTED
KETO PRODUCTS

Following you will find some selected books and supplies to support your Ketogenic journey, as with all other content of this book please consult first your health profesional before using any product on youself or administer to your AD patient.

Please note that each product description is followed by an exclusive purchase link (we apologize for the complicate format), please use such for the authors to earn a small sales comission via "affiliate marketing" (same price to you), which could help support ongoing efforts of research, attending conferences, and paper/book writing about this essential, often neglected, public health topic. Thank you very much!

Book: The Alzheimer's Antidote: Using a Low-Carb, High-Fat Diet to Fight Alzheimer's Disease, Memory Loss, and Cognitive Decline (Amy Berger, 2017). **Buy clicking here:** https://amzn.to/3bjR8PK

Book: The End of Alzheimer's: The First Program to Prevent and Reverse Cognitive Decline Hardcover (Dale Bredesen, 2017) **Buy clicking here:** https://amzn.to/2H77Cwt

Exogenous Ketones: As discussed these products are an excelent way to complement or facilitate supply of Ketones to a patient possibly whilst the diet is slowly being modified to match Ketogenic guideliness. **Buy clicking here:** https://amzn.to/39cXy1a

MCT Oil: As discussed possibly the simplest and most natural way to supplement an existing diet for an AD patient, do not overdo as could initialy cause digestive issues. MCT Oil is quickly processed by the liver and converted in Ketones. Try adding to coffe, tea (mix well) or salads. **Buy clicking here:** https://amzn.to/31DvEZB

Fat percentage scales: The best way to keep an eye in changing weight, muscle, water and far percentage composition is by means these type of scales, its important to keep monitoring bodily changes due to any dietary modification **Buy clicking here:** https://amzn.to/39cQ4ep

Keto sticks: The easiest and safest way to find out if you have reached the state of Ketosis, is using these sticks which react to an urine drop, changing color in a purple scale to indicate the precense and amount of discarded ketones (its perfectly normal for that to happen). **Buy clicking here:** https://amzn.to/2UvSgd1

Any questions or additional product recomendations please contact the authors at admin@curebyketo.com

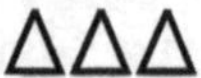

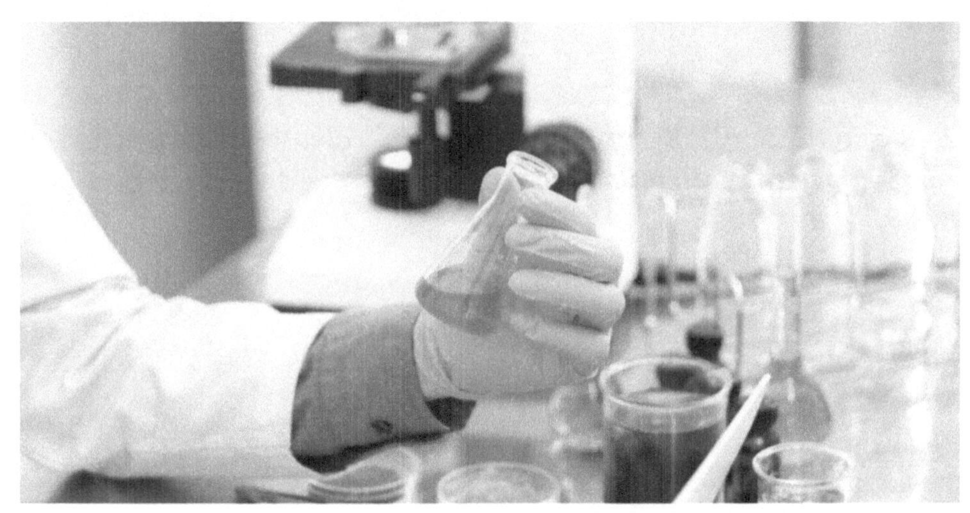

REFERENCES

We are aware the Internet is full of misleading, incomplete and even contraductory information. Therefore to fulfill the goal of this book becomming a serious and trustable source of information, the authors reviewed dozens of scientific papers, follows the list of major references utilized.

Dear reader: If you want to make suggestions about the content of this book, including error reports, improvements, or to suggest additional sources (i.e. research papers), please kindly contact the authors.

1.- Klaus W. Lange, Katharina M. Lange, Ewelina Stollberg, Yukiko Nakamura, el al:
Ketogenic diets and Alzheimer's disease (November 2016.)

http://bit.ly/3bnM7FB

LINK

2.- Sarah J. Morrill, Kelly J. Giba, *Ketogenic diet rescues cognition in ApoE4+ patient with mild Alzheimer's disease: A case study (January 2019)*

http://bit.ly/2ODZOXg

LINK

3.- Ana I. Rojo, Marta Pajares, Patricia Rada, Angel Nunez Alejo J., Nevado- Holgado, et al: *NRF2 deficiency replicates transcriptomic changes in Alzheimer's patients and worsens APP and TAU pathology*

http://bit.ly/2OwZ2LR

LINK

4.- Yoshihiro Kashiwaya, Takao Takeshima, Nozomi Mori, Kenji Nakashima*, Kieran Clarke†, and Richard L. Veech Corrections: *D-β -Hydroxybutyrate protects neurons in models of Alzheimer's and Parkinson's disease, (2000)*

http://bit.ly/31FwFQP

LINK

5.- Dariusz Włodarek: *Role of Ketogenic Diets in Neurodegenerative Diseases (Alzheimer's Disease and Parkinson's Disease), (Jan 2019)*

http://bit.ly/3bnPrR6

LINK

6.- Zhu TB, Zhang Z, Luo P, Wang SS, Peng Y, Chu SF, Chen NH: *Lipid metabolism in Alzheimer's disease, (November 2018) http://bit.ly/2vUUNTH*

LINK

7.- Suzanne Craft: *Effect of a Ketogenic Diet on Alzheimer's Disease Biomarkers and Symptoms "Brain Energy for Amyloid Transformation in AD (BEAT-AD)" Study (16 February 2018)*

http://bit.ly/3bpr1ae

LINK

8.- Stephen C. Cunnane, Alexandre Courchesne-Loyer, Val´erie St-Pierre, Camille Vandenberghe, Tyler Pierotti, M´elanie Fortier, Etienne Croteau, and Christian- Alexandre Castellano: *Can ketones compensate for deteriorating brain glucose uptake during aging? Implications for the risk and treatment of Alzheimer's disease, (2016).*

http://bit.ly/2vismyE

LINK

9.- Mary T. Newport: *MD, KETONES AS AN ALTERNATIVE FUEL FOR ALZHEIMER'S DISEASE AND OTHER DISORDERS, May 2014*

http://bit.ly/2H3wx4d

LINK

10.- Taylor, Matthew K., et al. *"Feasibility and Efficacy Data from a Ketogenic Diet Intervention in Alzheimer's Disease." Alzheimer's & Dementia: Translational Research & Clinical Interventions, vol. 4, 2018, pp. 28–36., doi:10.1016/j.trci.2017.11.002.*

http://bit.ly/376gbCA

LINK

ΔΔΔ